The
Bulletproof
Keto Diet

Lose Weight
and
Reboot Your Metabolism

Ron Kness

Published by:

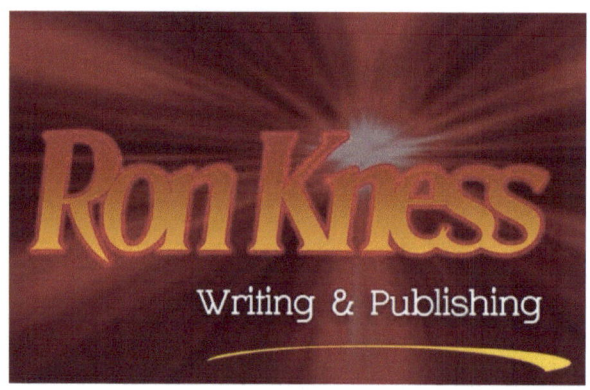

Ron Kness

San Tan Valley, AZ

United States of America

ISBN: 9781070181189

Sneak Peek

I don't know how many diets you've been through, but let me tell you, if you don't have the right mindset going in with this expertly-written Bulletproof Keto Diet or implement it the correct way, then chances are you're not going to succeed.

Having the right mindset

In fact, if you're like most people, your experience with diets in the past fit a very familiar pattern. First, you're all excited about the diet and sure enough, you follow the directions very closely.

Thanks to your careful dietary (and restricted) guidelines, and your eager compliance, you start losing a lot of pounds. So far so good, right? This keeps up for maybe a few more days or even a few more weeks. But sooner or later, the cravings kick in because of the food you have been denying yourself and pounds start coming back.

Next, things go from bad to worse. You start gaining more weight than when you began your diet. Isn't the whole point of going on a diet to lose weight? Sadly, most diets are gateways, believe it or not, to additional weight; talk about a frustrating situation.

One reason why people go through this all too familiar tragic pattern is because they don't have the right mindset. It doesn't matter which diet plan you adopt, without the right mindset, you are playing the game to lose.

Most diets are meant to be short-term. Maybe you want to lose a few pounds for an upcoming wedding or class reunion. But afterward you go back to your old eating habits and gain the weight back on. Why? Because your diet did not teach you how to eat healthy for the long-term; how to make your eating a healthy lifestyle change.

With the Bulletproof Keto Diet, your mindset must be that it is a lifestyle change and a healthy eating plan that you can live on for the rest of your life. You can't view it as a short-term fix for a long-term problem.

Implementing the Bulletproof Keto Diet

The other thing different with this diet, besides it being a healthy lifestyle change instead of just another short-term diet, is how it is implemented. With most other diets, you are restricted from eating certain food groups. In the beginning, this will work, but eventually your body will demand the food you have been denying it. As mentioned before, you'll start to have cravings … and we know from experience, cravings win out every time.

But the Bulletproof Keto Diet is implemented differently. Instead of *replacing* food, it *displaces* food. Let me explain…

In the beginning on this diet you don't deny yourself any of the food you like. You cut down on those foods and instead add in the low carb/high fat food on the Keto diet.

As you settle into this diet, your food tastes will begin to change – literally your taste buds change from wanting your old food to wanting the food on the keto diet. Over time, you'll slowly and naturally gravitate toward keto food (https://www.amazon.com/gp/product/1091823219) and less of the food you used to like. By doing it this natural way, you eliminate cravings.

It's really important to focus on enjoying your food. It shouldn't be an ordeal. This is not some sort of punishment or a situation where you feel that you are denying yourself. Instead, the keto diet should be a celebration of taste. It all really boils down to enjoying your food according to keto rules.

With the right mindset - that this is a lifestyle change - and that you are going to displace food instead of replacing it, this healthy eating plan will work for you just as it has worked for many others including celebrities, athletes and musicians.

If you are looking for permanent weight loss, you owe it to yourself to buy this Bulletproof Keto Diet book. It is like no other one out there right now. What do you have to lose?

Contents

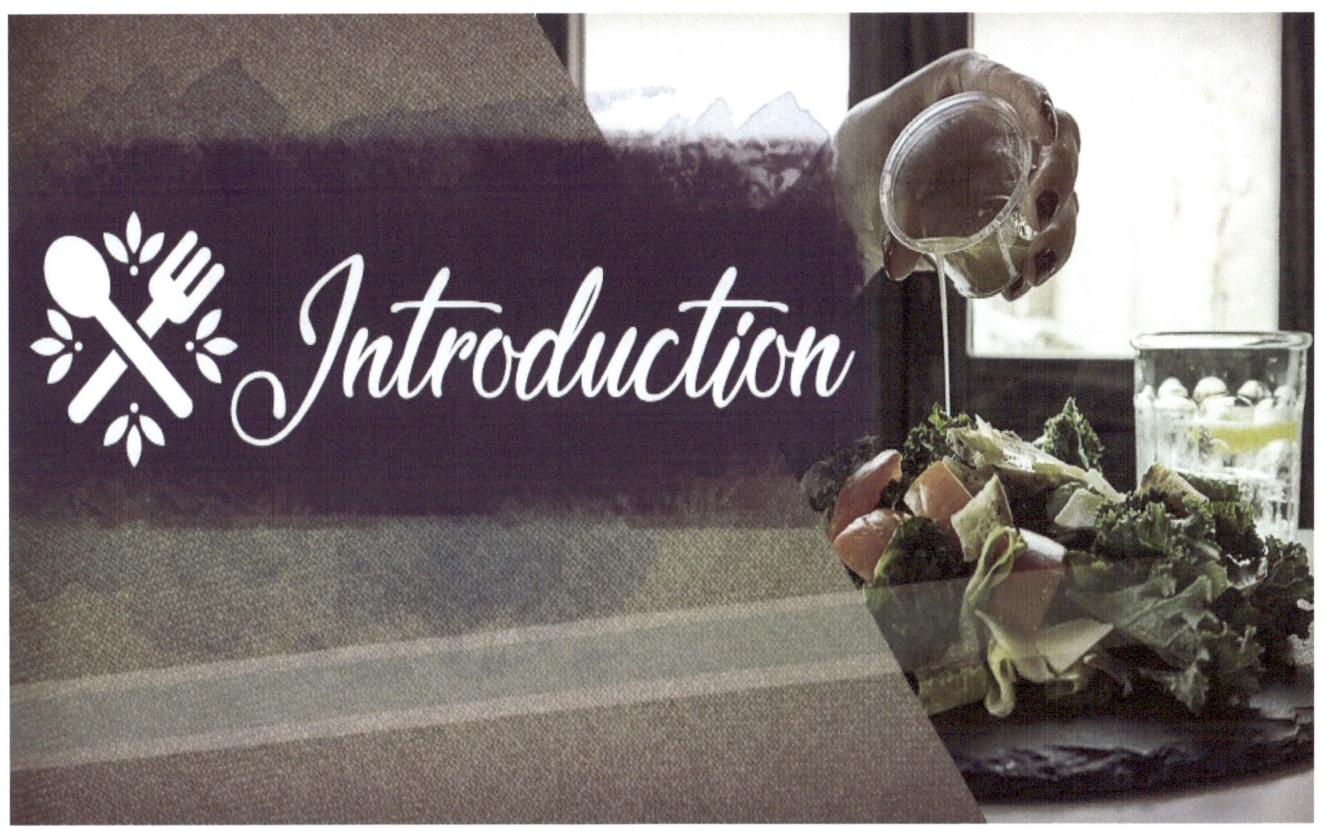

Introduction

If you're reading this book, you probably are a veteran of several diets. I can't say I blame you because you are not alone. In fact, millions of Americans try one diet after another only to end up in the same place. Actually, too many of us go on diet after diet and we get heavier and heavier each time we try.

It's bad enough that a lot of these diets are unable to keep the weight off but once you get off the diet, you gain more pounds. It's a very frustrating situation and a lot of people have basically thought that outside of surgery, losing weight on a sustainable basis is pretty much a pipedream.

You're in luck. It turns out, according to recent research, dietary fat (https://www.amazon.com/gp/product/B0120OZLN4) has actually gotten a bad rap. Based on these recent analyses, the real culprit for America's exploding waistline is none other than sugar. You heard that right.

The old idea of eating a lot of fruits, starchy food and starchy vegetables is actually making you sick. It leads to inflammation; it increases the chances of developing certain types of cancer; and it inflames the system so much that it can put people at risk of cardiovascular diseases.

By loading up on eggs, avocados, and other high-fat, low-carb foods, you can live healthier while losing weight on a sustainable basis. The key is achieving ketosis. Don't get scared of the term. Your body can take only two forms of energy. Either it uses up the sugar in your bloodstream or it takes in fat in the form of chemical compounds produced by your liver called ketones.

When people achieve ketosis, they not only lose weight, but they get a nice burst of energy; they think more clearly; their skin improves and a whole long list of tremendous health benefits. If you are looking for a great way to adopt the keto diet and recalibrate your metabolism for sustainable weight loss, you are reading the right book.

In this book, I'm going to step you through the basics of a keto diet so as to maximize your chances of success. Please understand that this book is a framework. In other words, I'm not going to make you stick to a rigid system like a typical diet book.

This book is a framework. You basically work with your existing diet and you switch gradually over to a ketogenic diet and you stay there. This way, you experience less psychological internal resistance to your lifestyle change. This is less a diet book and more a lifestyle-modification book – something shown over and over as to what is needed for permanent and sustainable weight loss. This is the same diet plan famous celebrities, athletes and musicians use to lose weight and get fit. And now it is available for you to use to get the same results.

Make no mistake, if you want the pounds to go and you want them to remain gone, you have to change your lifestyle. Stop going on diet after diet. The constant cycle of losing weight, gaining it back, losing it over and over is super hard on your body physically not to mention what it does to you emotionally. Instead, change your attitude about certain foods and change your lifestyle. It can be done. This book written by an expert in the field will teach you how to do it.

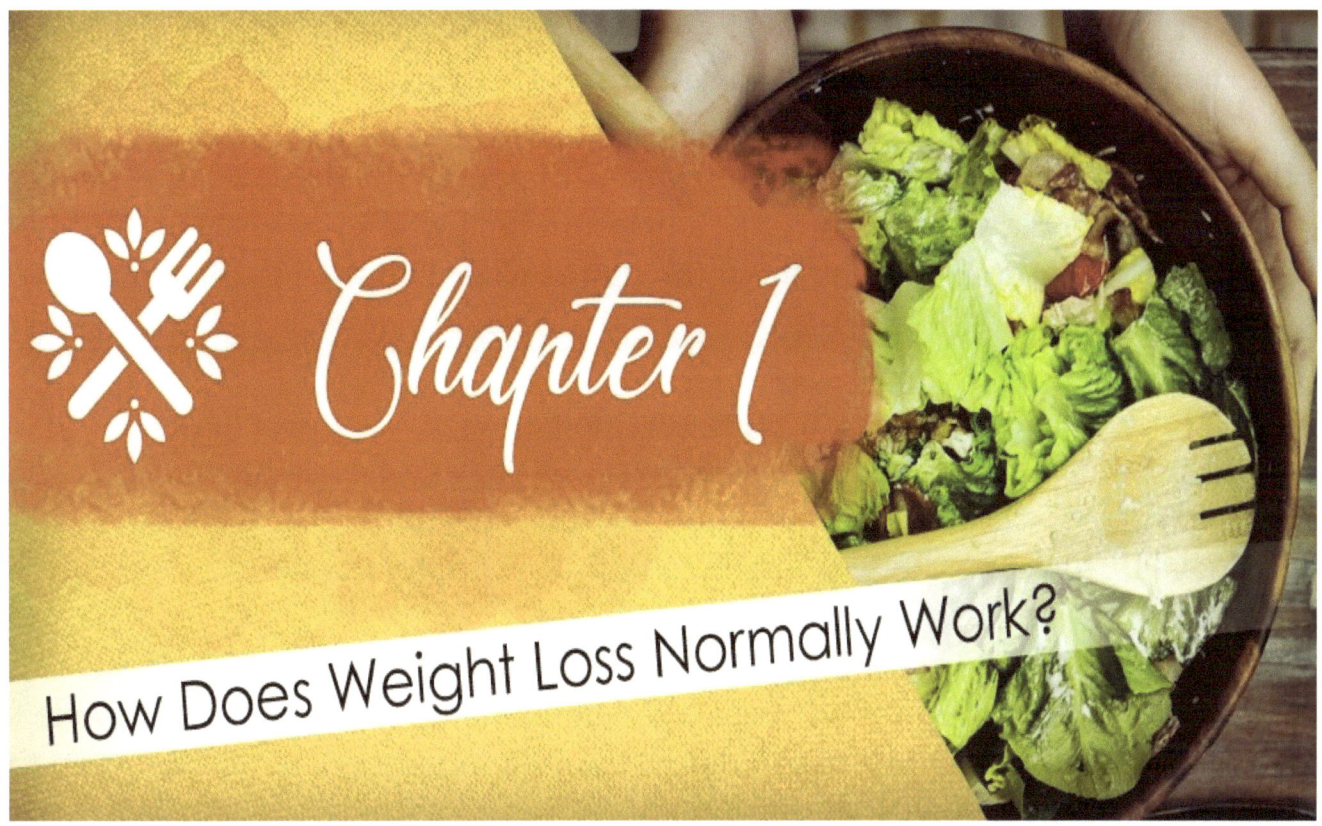

Chapter 1 – How Does Weight Loss Normally Work?

What if I told you that weight loss is actually pretty straightforward. You might be thinking that I've lost my mind. If you are like most people who have been struggling with their weight, "simple" is not the first word to enter your mind when asked to describe dieting.

It's easy to be frustrated about weight loss. A lot of people have a tough time losing weight and keeping the pounds off. However, when you look at human metabolism with a big picture of you, it's actually pretty straightforward.

In fact, it can be reduced to a simple mathematical formula: calories in verses calories out. When you try to lose weight, you really only have 2 options. It may seem like there are tons of weight loss options and systems out there, but it really all boils down to these 3 methods. Everything else is a variation of these 3 methods or categories.

Method #1: Eat fewer calories but burn the same amount of energy.

In any given day, you are already burning calories. That's right! Just by simply reading this book, you are burning calories. In fact, when you wake up and you breathe and digest food throughout the day as well as pump blood, you are burning calories.

The bottom line is if your body does anything at all, it requires energy. In other words, it's burning calories. This is called your passive calorie burn rate. If you were to eat less calories than the amount of energy your body needs to function every single day, your body is forced to look at your stored energy.

In other words, it starts eating your fat and, eventually, your muscle tissues. That's how it works. Your body has to get enough energy somehow to be able to do what it needs to do on a day to day basis. When there is a deficit between the number of calories you eat and the amount of energy you burn, your body starts to burn up fat.

Before you know it, you start weighing less and you start looking better and better.

Method #2: Eat the same number of calories but burn energy at a higher rate.

You can also choose to flip the script. When people decide to go to the gym or start doing physical exercises daily, this is what they're doing. They eat the same amount of food, but they increase their physical activities.

Please understand that you don't have to overdo it. You don't have to do something dramatic in terms of your physical exertion levels. By simply just walking around the block or walking a longer distance from the parking lot to your office or school, you can burn more energy.

Again, the same process takes place. When you eat the same amount of calories but your body burns more energy, it's going to start looking for other sources of energy. It starts to burn fat and then, eventually, it starts to burn muscle.

The end result is the same. You start losing weight.

Method #3: Burn the weight loss candle from both ends.

This is a no brainer. Since you know that you can lose weight just by eating less calories while burning the same amount of energy or you can eat the same amount of calories while burning more energy, why not do both? That's the third option.

Again, self explanatory.

In terms of a big picture view, this is how weight loss normally works. It's all about calories in, calories out. As simple as this may sound, people have a tough time doing this because of the standard American diet.

Now, please understand that thanks to modern food technology and transport systems, the standard American diet did not remain in the confines of the United States. If you are middle class pretty much all over the world, chances are you have adopted the standard American diet and it's making you fatter and fatter.

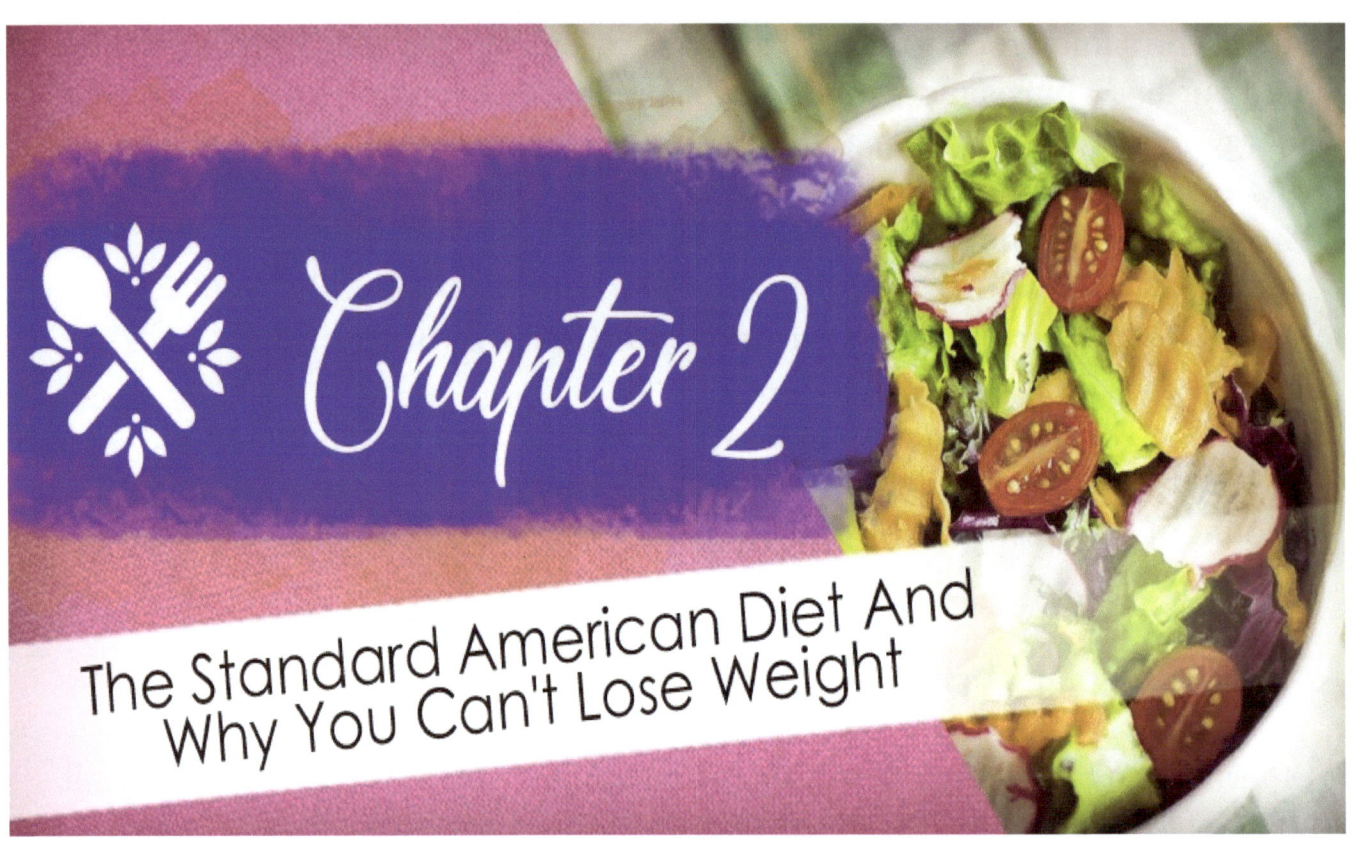

Chapter 2 – The Standard American Diet and Why You Can't Lose Weight

The standard American diet seems pretty innocuous at first glance. I mean, who has a problem with eating a certain amount of protein and a certain amount of carbohydrates in the form of fruits and vegetables and grains and small amount of fat, if at all?

It's probably been drilled into your head for over several years that this is the healthy way to go. Nobody can really blame you for thinking otherwise. But what if I told you that the standard American diet, with its heavy focus on protein and carbohydrates, is actually making you sick and making you fat?

Carbohydrates and the problem with insulin

Whenever you have more than 12 to 20 grams of carbohydrates in your diet, insulin is going to be an issue. Normally, insulin is a good thing.

Insulin, after all, is the hormone that unlocks your body's cells so it lets in the sugar in your bloodstream. Once your cells absorb the sugar, it then converts it into energy.

Well here's the problem with insulin. It has a dark side. When insulin is in your system, your body uses blood sugar for fuel. This means it's not burning fat. In fact, insulin has the effect of locking your fat cells so none of that energy gets out.

Your body is blocked from using fat as energy. That spare tire you're walking around with will remain with you until and unless you deal with insulin. Reduce insulin and your body starts burning fat for fuel. It's that simple.

The problem is the standard American diet has so much carbohydrates that people starts suffering from the excesses of insulin. Not only do they have spikes in insulin levels which leads to them feeling hungry throughout the day, a high-carb diet also inflames your system.

The truth about fat loss

If you want to burn belly fat or you just want to lose a lot of weight, you have to focus on controlling your insulin levels. It doesn't get any simpler than that. When insulin is in the picture, it's going to block off your fat cells and your body is not going to burn fat for energy. There's no chance of it doing that.

Chapter 3 – The Keto Alternative

Thankfully, there is an alternative to using blood sugar for cellular energy. You can use fat. Now this flies in the face of all the health guidance you probably have heard throughout the years. I remember, since I was a kid hearing again and again, that fat is evil and saturated fat is bad for you. That's all I heard.

Health authorities and advisory boards were saying that I should load up on mashed potatoes, rice, vegetables, fruits, so on and so forth. It turns out that it's the other way around.

The real health emergency in America and elsewhere is the high amount of sugar (read: simple carbohydrates) in our diets. It's the sugar that's making us sick. It's the sugar that is inflaming us. It's the sugar that is positioning us to developing certain types of cancer later on. Who knew?

The ketosis alternative

If your body doesn't use sugar for energy, its only other alternative is to use fat. Your liver metabolizes fat in the form of ketones. These biochemical compounds are absorbed by your cells and transformed into energy.

Ketosis explained

Ketosis refers to the biochemical process your body goes through when it starts burning fat for energy. Normally, your body burns sugar in your bloodstream as well as the sugar stored in your liver and muscles. Worst comes to worst, your body would turn protein into sugar courtesy of your liver.

When you burn fat for energy, your pancreas does not release insulin since there is no sugar involved. This means that you feel fuller longer. You're no longer eating throughout the day like you would if you were on a standard carbohydrate rich diet.

The reason why a lot of people gain weight is because they can't stop eating throughout the day. This is due to the fact that their insulin peaks and crashes several times during the day. These peaks and crashes trigger your brain to feel hungry. Your body starts sending out hunger signals and you can't help but eat.

Obviously, the more calories you eat and the less calories you burn or if you burn calories at the same rate as you normally do, you end up storing those excess calories into fat. You let go of all of that when you switch over to fat. Your body burns fat instead of sugar, so you feel fuller for a longer period of time.

No, you're not going to die with ketosis! One of the most common misconceptions about going on a keto diet is that you end up polluting your blood with ketone bodies to the point that you die. This is a myth. Usually, the people who develop this condition called ketoacidosis are people who cannot naturally produce insulin.

In other words, people most prone to ketoacidosis are Type 1 diabetics. There's a good chance you're not a Type 1 diabetic, but if you are then you should not use this diet. Most people aren't.

This is why you shouldn't worry about developing ketoacidosis because at some level, your body is still producing insulin. It really can't go completely off insulin.

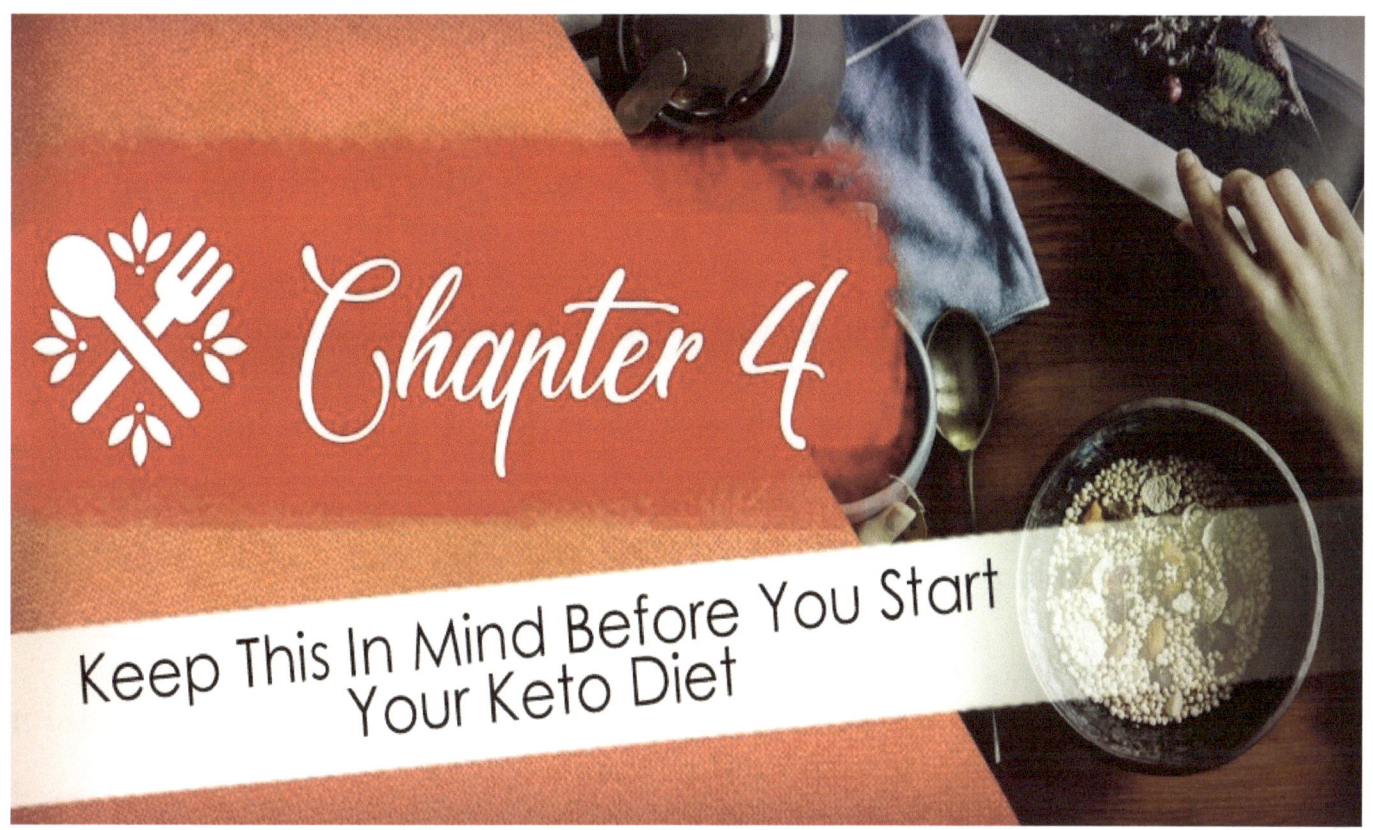

Chapter 4 – Keep This In Mind Before You Start Your Keto Diet

If you want your keto diet to be a success, you need to wrap your mind around what I'm about to share with you. If you neglect this chapter, chances are you are not going to stay on the keto diet for long. There's a high likelihood that you're probably going to look at your keto diet as just another thing that you've tried so you can lose weight.

In other words, it's just another diet to you. Last time I checked, that is a losing strategy. Keep an open mind and focus on the following.

Change your lifestyle instead of going on another diet

Don't look at the keto diet as just another diet option. I know that I used the term "keto diet", but if you look at it closely, it's actually something bigger than a simple decision to switch from one class of foods to another.

It's actually a lifestyle change. You're going to change your taste buds. Previously, you may not have much of a preference for oily foods. But once you make that switch, it becomes harder to switch back. Your perspective has changed along with your tastes.

Think long term

The keto diet is actually a long term strategy. It's not something that you try because you have to lose weight for your high school reunion. It's not something that you get on because you just want to lose weight by a certain date.

It is a long term program because it reprograms your taste buds and, ultimately, changes your relationship with food and your attitude towards eating. If you think along these lines, your chances of succeeding with the keto diet increases tremendously.

A lot of Americans go through this process where they go on a diet and they lose weight. They gain the weight back and they weigh more after a few months. They then go on a diet, then go on another diet and repeat the process again and again.

Once enough time passes, they end up massively overweight. They didn't pack on the extra pounds because they wanted to. But that's where they end up. This is because they don't think long term. They don't think in terms of lifestyle change.

Instead, they look at a weight loss program as simply another diet. Stop doing that! It has proven to those who have tied that it does not work, so why try another diet just like the ones that have failed you and others before?

Believe that the keto lifestyle works

I cannot even begin to tell you how many times people have been counseled regarding weight loss and after nodding their heads for what seemed like hours, they ask, "Honestly, do you think it's going to work for me?"

This reflects the love/hate relationship too many people have with weight loss programs. At the end of the day, they believe that it's not going to work for them.

It is no surprise that with this mindset, people are able to only lose weight initially at best.

That's the best they could do because ultimately, their lack of trust and belief in the system eats away at their resolve. Eventually, they believe that the system really doesn't work and they're back to where they began. Sad. Totally unnecessary.

If you're going to adopt the keto diet, you have to believe that this lifestyle works. Period. And to help you believe, read some of the testimonials. Look at the people that have lost a tremendous amount of weight using this system. Believe that it works. And if you know that celebrities use this diet with the limited time they have available, it works … otherwise they would not be doing it.

Otherwise, your lack of belief and trust is going to erode your efforts at implementing it … just like the last time and the time before and the … I think you get the picture. Eventually, you're going to slow down and the pounds will come rushing back. The worst part? You did it to yourself. And you didn't have to!

Believe that YOU can do it

It's one thing to believe that the keto lifestyle works for other people. It's another thing to believe that it works for you. If you want the keto diet to truly deliver its claims, believe that you can do it. Believe that when you get on it, you will benefit from it.

There's really no point in thinking that something works for other people. So what? That's them. We're talking about you. So, make sure that you believe that this can work for you. The good news is if other people can do it, why can't you? The truth is you can!

Aren't you any less entitled to losing all that weight? Can't you benefit the same way as other people including many famous people in Hollywood and other places? Don't think, for whatever reason, that you're unique and special and can not lose weight through systems that benefit other people. Believe that you can make it work. Having a mindset of success is so powerful!

The bottom line: If other people can do it, you can do it too. As the old saying goes, the proof is in the pudding. All these keto testimonials as well as the personal "before and after" pictures that you see all over the internet involving the keto diet, they're absolutely true.

They work for people. Keto was working yesterday, it's working today, it will continue to work in the future. Why? Because it involves a biological change that functions the same today as it did yesterday and will be the same tomorrow. Now the question is are you going to look at what happened to those people and accept that it can also happen to you?

If you have a tough time believing that you can achieve what other people have achieved with the keto diet, they you just have to admit that you're giving yourself excuses not to try. That's the bottom line. You're coming up with one justification after another and one excuse after another not to try. That's what's really going on.

Get your mind right before you start your keto diet

You need to go through all the steps above and everything must line up. If you don't get into this with the right mindset, chances are you will end up sabotaging yourself. There's a high likelihood that you will eventually stumble, lose motivation and go back to your old eating patterns.

I understand that you're frustrated with your weight. I understand that you want to change. But no change is possible until and unless you change your mindset. In this chapter, I've laid out the mental changes that you need to go through so you can tackle the keto diet with the right attitude. Next let's look at how to actually implement those changes.

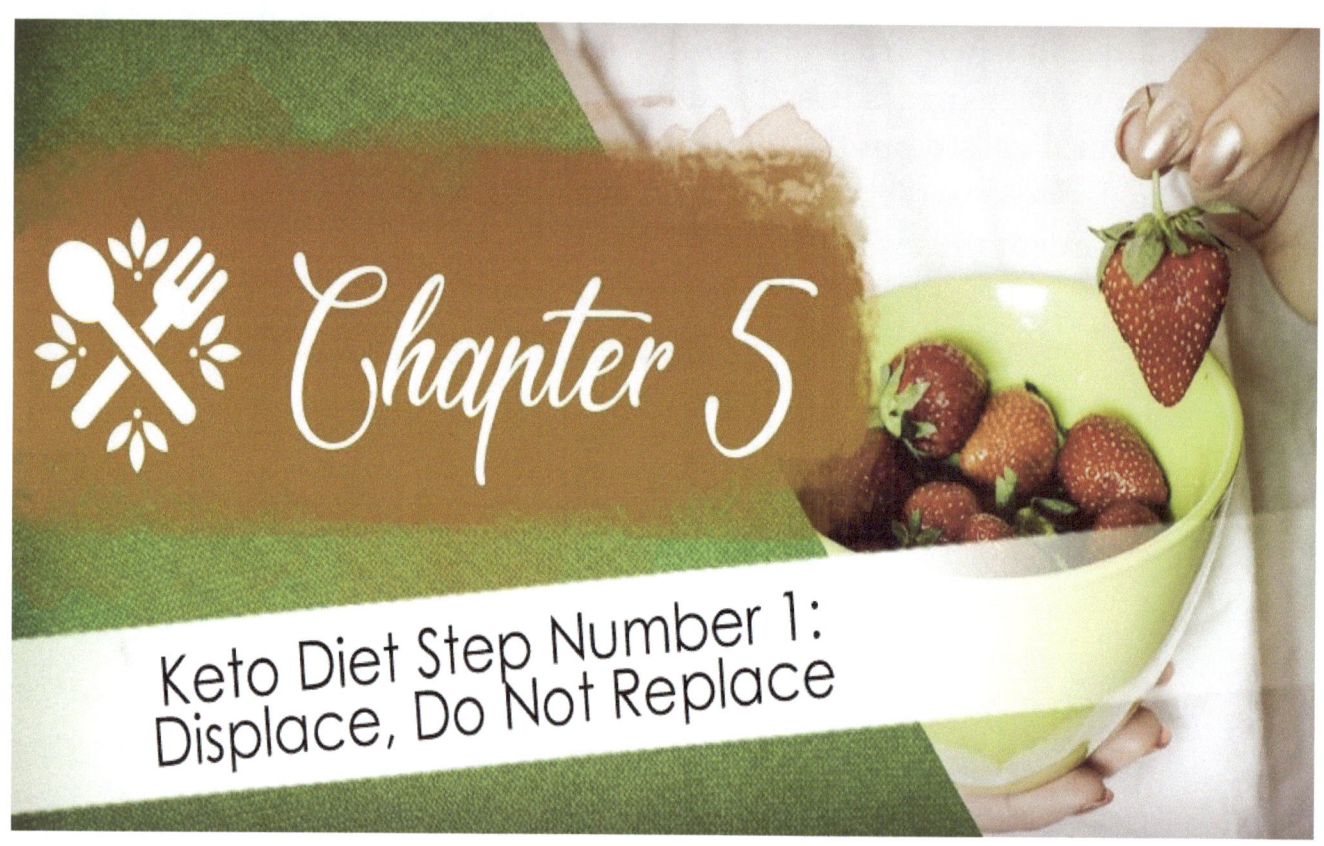

Chapter 5 – Keto Diet Step Number 1: Displace, Do Not Replace

One of the most common problems I've seen people run into again and again with diets is they use a scorched earth policy. For example, if somebody is loading up on starch, they basically replace all the meat and all the eggs and fatty food they have been eating with just starch.

They have this black and white, either or, all or nothing mindset. Now you may be thinking that this is a good thing. You may be thinking that this indicates commitment and a firm decision to make a change. That might be true.

The problem is when you go through such an abrupt change, your body starts to push back. At first, it's not all that noticeable. But eventually, your mind and your body starts pulling you back to your old eating habits; this pull is called cravings and they will win out every time.

You have to understand that we're all creatures of habit. We've grown accustomed to certain things. We adopt certain lifestyles because they meet our needs at a very deep level. Your weight and your eating patterns are reflections of your personal habits and your chosen lifestyle.

As you probably already know, changing habits is not very easy. As a matter of fact, it takes between 21 and 30 days to make a change into a habit. It's definitely not something that you take on lightly. It is no surprise, given this background that a lot of people who just abruptly change their diets end up going back to their old eating patterns.

All that weight they've lost initially in the early stages of the diet come back. Worse yet, people get heavier. They end up in a worse place than when they started. This is due to the fact that they triggered their system for a serious backlash later on.

Just because it didn't happen when you switched over to your new diet doesn't mean it's not going to happen. It's like trapping heat in a volcano. It's only a matter of time until that volcano blows its top. This is exactly what happens to a lot of people switching from one lifestyle to another and one diet to another.

It doesn't matter whether you've adopted the paleo diet, the south beach diet, the Atkins diet or any other kind of weight loss program. Eventually, you go back to your old eating habits.

The number 1 reason why people cannot sustain their new diet

Why do people end up where they begin? The most common problem with diets is that people choose to *replace* instead of *blending in new ingredients*. For example, if you used to eating a lot of rice, mashed potatoes, white bread, pasta and other starchy staples, you probably would want to clean out your pantry once you switch over to a paleo or other high fat low carb diet.

This is a common tendency with a lot of people adopting new diets. They simply just want to turn their back on their old eating patterns because they can see the benefits the new diet brings to the table. They've seen before and after pictures of people losing a ridiculous amount of weight.

They can see how good people look after shedding all that fat. They can't wait to just stop what they're eating and eat new food. I understand why people are excited. I was excited too. But after seeing myself in worse shape after my diet than when I began, it dawned on me.

I began to realize that the reason why I keep coming back to where I started is because is sought to replace all my food choices. I used a scorched earth policy. I would go from eating fruits and vegetables to eating only eggs, avocados and other fatty foods. After all, I've gone keto.

You can say the same for paleo and other diets out there. The problem is this is not sustainable. I was only able to stay on the keto diet when I started to displace food items. What does this mean? Instead of replacing high carb items on my meal plans, I added high fat items to my diet.

Eventually, I started to lose my taste for high carb foods. They got displaced by more and more high fat items on my meal plans. Add. Do not subtract. Displace. Do not replace.

It's all in your head

Remember, the reason why you are displacing and not replacing and adding instead of cutting out large chunks of your meal plan is because you're trying to work with your psychology. When you start taking out dishes from your meal plan, your mind starts feeling left behind. Deep down inside, you start to feel that you're denying yourself. You feel like you are losing something.

I'm sure I don't need to remind you that one of the most powerful human impulses is the fear of loss or getting left behind. This is the reason why people who live in certain neighborhoods automatically get the urge to buy the same car as their neighbor once their neighbor rolls around in a new set of wheels.

I've seen this happen quite a bit. It only takes one neighbor to buy a new top of the line Mercedes Benz or BMW to get other neighborhoods to want to buy the same kind of car. The same applies to clothes. The same applies to food and lifestyle.

We don't like to get left behind. We don't like to feel like we are denying ourselves. This is exactly the kind of mindset you trigger when you choose to replace certain food choices from your diet on a wholesale basis. Don't do it!

Instead, keep adding ketogenic meal items to your diet. Eventually, you will reach a point where your taste buds have switched over to a fat preference. You're no longer craving sweets. You no longer feel like you can't go a day without carbohydrates. That's when these carb items start dropping from your meal plan.

However, it has to take place gradually. You can't force it.

Focus more on ketogenic meals

As mentioned before (at least a couple of times now) you get used to eating keto friendly meals, your taste buds begin to change. At first it may seem like it may be hard going for you. After all, who can eat eggs day after day? If you're like most Americans, you probably don't really have much of a craving for avocado on a daily basis. I'm probably not like most Americans in this aspect in that my wife and I eat about 5 avocados per week and eggs three times per week.

Eventually, it becomes routine to you and you start craving more ketogenic items and start forgetting about your old sweet tooth. Still, you have to do this gradually. You can't shock your system. The moment you shock your system, be prepared for the back lash because your body is sure to put up a fight and it will win .. every .. single .. time.

It may not do it immediately, but eventually, it will undermine you. Eventually, it will get the upper hand. Before you know it, you're back to eating what you used to eat before you adopted your keto diet.

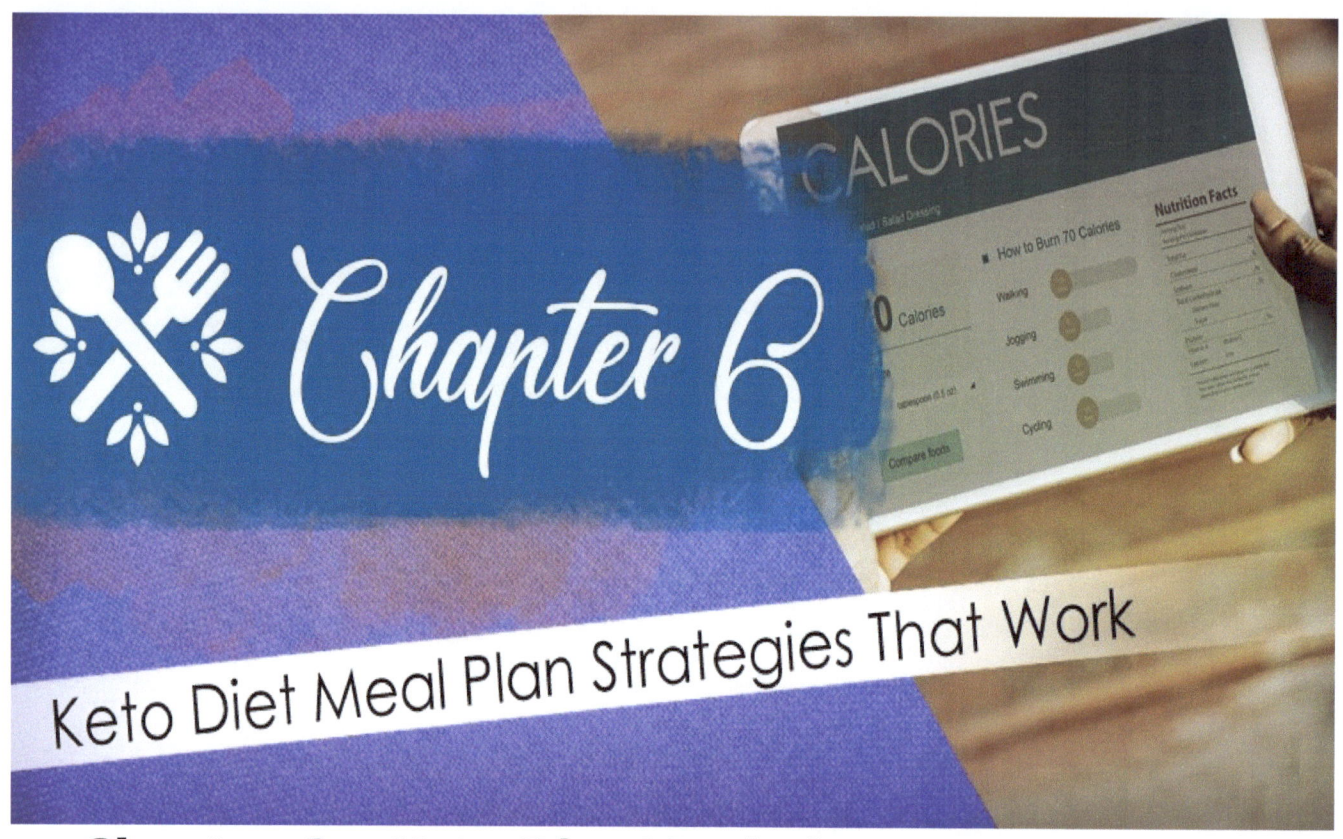

Chapter 6 – Keto Diet Meal Plan Strategies That Work

As I have mentioned in the previous chapter, if you don't have the right mindset coming in, there's a high chance you are going to fail with your keto diet.

However to be fair, if you are mentally unprepared for your weight loss journey, you probably will fail with most other diets too ... probably as you have done in the past. Don't think that this is limited to keto.

Your lack of mental preparation may mean you may have certain emotional vulnerabilities which can translate to you getting off your keto diet sooner rather than later. Thankfully, there are certain strategies that you can use if you have the right mindset.

Having the right "weight loss mindset" is essential. It is non-negotiable. There is no getting around it. This is why I suggest that before you go any further, review Chapter 5 again thoroughly. Your mind must be in the right place before starting this diet.

Remember weight loss is as much about mentally as it is physically ... even more so.

With that said, here are some key strategies that would help you transition to a keto diet and stick with it.

Quick Note

Transitioning to keto is actually easy. Seriously.

When you're beginning any kind of diet, you would be pumped up. You would be excited about getting started because you know that it benefits a lot of people. You have seen the results other people got so you can't wait to try it yourself.

Getting started is not the problem. Getting pumped up, getting excited, and getting ready are all awesome. The problem is sticking to it.

This is why you need the right mindset and the right meal plan strategies. Please focus on the following.

Focus on Fatty Food that Fits Your Taste

One of the most commonly recommended high-fat foods for people starting out on keto is avocado.

Well, it's easy to see why avocado is a "usual suspect." It is high in fiber and it's loaded with fat. What's not to love?

The problem is, if you don't have a particular taste for avocado, it might seem like you are nibbling on a piece of wax. It takes some getting used to. Personally, my wife and I enjoy it cut up and placed on top of a salad.

Most people usually mix avocado with something else. Either they turn it into guacamole and enjoy it with Mexican dishes, or they turn it into some sort of ice cream.

Now, you know that on a keto diet, you cannot enjoy regular ice cream. This snack is loaded with sugar and milk, which has lactose.
So, you're stuck with a plain avocado.

There is a workaround to this. Focus on fatty foods that already have the taste profile you already prefer. In other words, stick with what you know.

If you already prefer certain foods like pork rinds or other oily, salty snacks, then load up on them. This is no time to acquire new tastes.

Remember, as I have mentioned in Chapter 5, the secret to transitioning to keto and sticking with it successfully over a sustained period of time is displacement, not replacement.

When you are trying to discover a new taste or trying to readjust your taste buds to accommodate new tastes, you are replacing.

Don't fool yourself into thinking that you are displacing your old meal plan. No. You are replacing. Bad strategy.

Sooner or later, something will get knocked loose and you will go back to your old eating habits. The better approach is to focus on fatty food that already fits your taste.

The good news is, we already have these. A lot of people who are not on a keto diet think that these are guilty pleasures. They think that they only should eat these dishes or snacks from time to time.

Well, when you switch over to a keto diet, your wish is fulfilled: you can eat those items pretty much every day. Isn't that good news?

Focus on fatty foods that already have the taste profile you desire.

Shoot to Feel Fuller for a Longer Period of Time

When you eat anything throughout the day, eat strategically. Say to yourself, "When I load up on this type of food, is it going to fill me up for a longer period of time?"

If you don't know what I'm getting at, think about the times when you used to eat apples as snacks. Sure, apples are light snacks, they're loaded with vitamins, but sooner rather than later, you're going to get hungry again. This is due to the fact that apples have sugar.

Now, if you replace apples with chocolate bars or candy bars or cookies, the same thing applies, but on a worse scale. You find yourself snacking throughout the day because of your blood sugar's roller coaster ride.

Once you switch over to a keto system, be strategic about what you eat. When you displace that apple with, let's say, a teaspoon of cream cheese, you feel fuller longer because the oil in your system is processed by your body differently. Your body sends different hunger signals to your brain and vice versa when you're eating fatty foods.

This is why it's crucial that you be as strategic as possible in your snacks. Instead of just grabbing anything to snack on, eat macadamia nuts. Those things are loaded with oil and your body can definitely tell. You feel fuller for a longer period of time.

Eventually Cut Out All Soda

By "all," I mean all.

A lot of people are thinking, "Well, I can go on a keto diet and cut out regular soda and hang on to diet drinks." These are soft drinks that are advertised as zero calories.

Well, first of all, they are not zero calories. Under U.S. labeling guidelines, they contain few enough calories that they can be pass as "zero calorie drinks" as far a nutritional labeling and advertising ... but they are not zero calories.

Also, recent studies have shown that people who drink diet colas actually have a shorter life expectancy. I know, it's shocking. It definitely shocked me. In fact, I got so stunned I swore off all sodas across the board.

It doesn't matter whether they are regular soda loaded with sugar, or high fructose corn syrup and other nasty junk, or they are the zero-calorie or low-calorie variety, I'm completely off them. And I suggest you do the same.

I understand that if you drink a lot of soda, it's going to be very hard to go cold turkey. Believe me, I can empathize. It took me a few false starts myself to finally get off the soda train.

This is why it's a good idea to follow one of the principles that I have laid out in Chapter 6: displace, do not replace.

In accordance with this piece of advice, eventually, cut out all soda. The key here is "eventually." This means that you must start today with zero soda as your eventual goal.

It doesn't have to be bold. It doesn't have to be dramatic. You're not trying to impress anybody, you're not trying to be a hero, but you must start today and gradually cut down.

If you do it gradually, it's actually much easier than you think. But if you were to go cold turkey, that's going to be a little bit of a problem because of the dynamics that I have described earlier in this book.

Your body will put up a fight. Your body is used to doing things a certain way. Your body has grown accustomed to certain patterns, and believe me, it's going to push back.

Sooner or later, you will find yourself doing the same things as before. Before you know it, you will be eating the same stuff as before.

So, don't do things that way. There's no need for some sort of black and white change.

Again, you're not trying to impress anybody. You're not trying to put on a show. Instead, you want to adopt something that will stick.

Eventually Cut Out Grain-Based Snacks

Let me be completely honest with you. One of the biggest hassles with adopting a keto diet involves snacks.

A lot of the snacks available out there are grain-based. It doesn't matter what you're into. Maybe you're into corn chips, corn flakes, puffed snacks, rice cakes, potato chips, the whole nine yards.

When you look at the common laundry list of snack items in the United States and elsewhere, they have one common denominator, for the most part. I am, of course, talking about grains.

It doesn't matter whether that grain is rice or corn, or it involves a starchy vegetable like potato. They're all loaded with starch. They're all off limits to you if you switch to a keto diet.

This is why it's a good idea to eventually cut down on grain-based snacks as you load up on fatty nuts like walnuts or macadamia.

Peanuts are off limits. Peanuts are not going to get you to where you want to go as far as your keto diet is concerned. Stick to high fat "bombs" like macadamia and walnuts.

This is a little bit tricky because, normally, macadamia nuts and walnuts are often packaged with chocolate or something sweet. You're going to have to make the adjustment to these nuts in their pure form.

The good news is that you probably already have a taste for them if you have had macadamia and walnuts as part of some sort of mixed nuts package. Load up on these.

Slowly Cut Out Milk-Based Snacks

Milk is a very touchy subject for a lot of people. A lot of individuals switching over to keto can easily make do without soda. Many are able to make the transition to a grain-free snack system with very little resistance. The problem is, once they try to cut out milk and dairy-based products, that's when they get a little antsy.

This is why I suggest that you slowly cut down. I'm not talking about eventually, I'm not talking about a fast withdrawal system, but just slowly cut out milk-based snacks and meal items.

It really all boils down to pacing yourself in line with your changing tastes. This is definitely not something that you can rush.

Keep the meal plan strategies above in mind. Make sure you try all of them. If you're having a tough time with one, keep at it.

Again, there's no need to be a hero. There's no need to just take one giant leap. You're not trying to prove anything to anybody.

What's important here is that you're able to stick to the changes that you have made. A little bit of incremental change can go a long way.

Some people adjust very quickly. Others need a little bit more time. Just figure out which one you are and just stick to the plan of action.

Eventually, your body will get used to it. Eventually, your taste buds will adjust.

If you are interested in a Keto Diet Cookbook this is a good one.
https://www.amazon.com/gp/product/1091823219

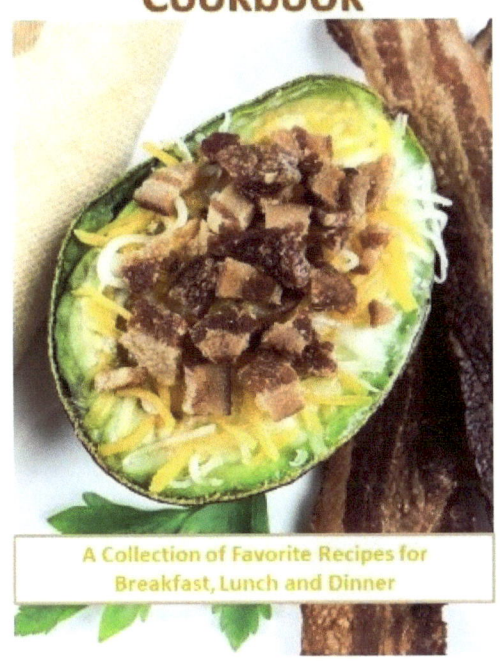

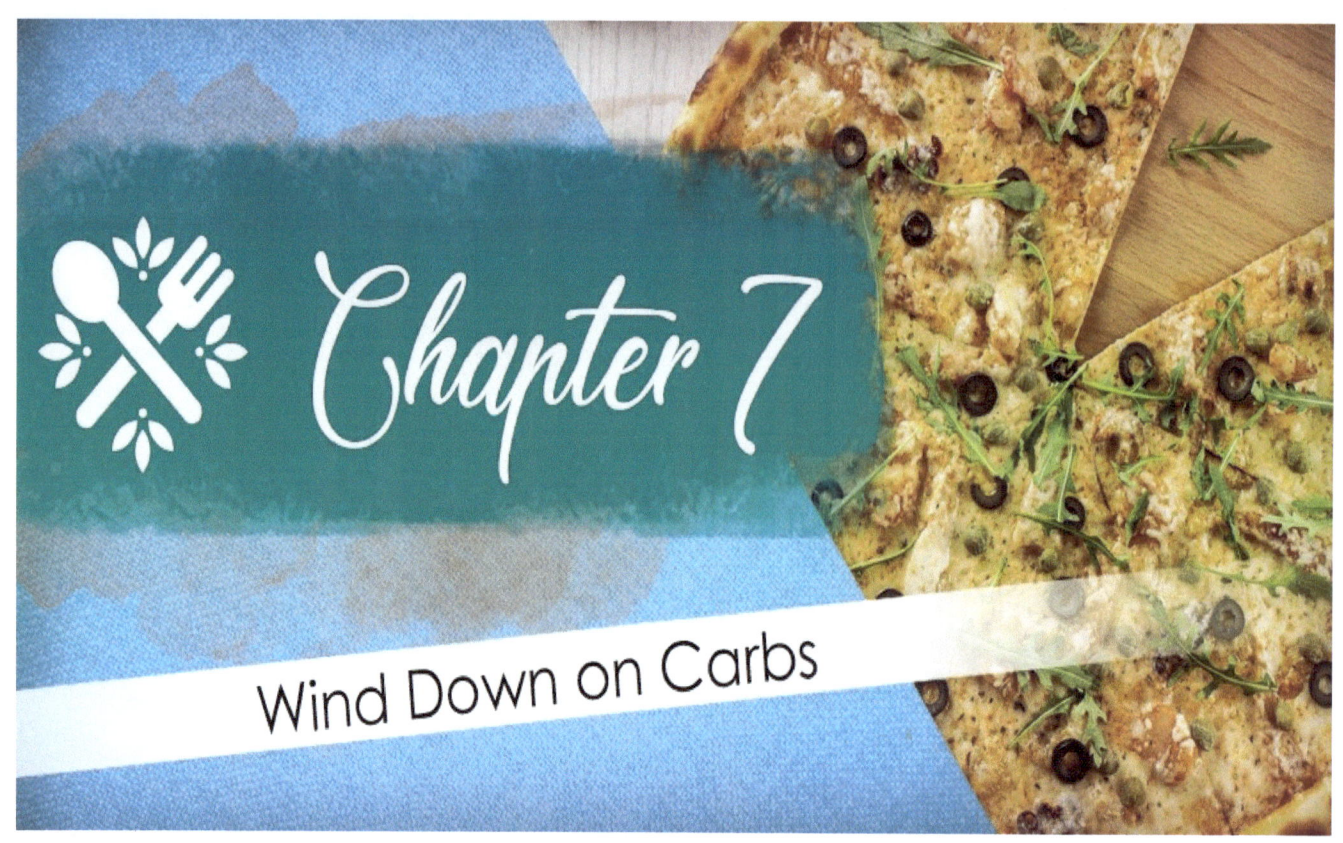

Chapter 7 – Wind Down on Carbs

By this point, you have gotten used to eating keto foods. Again, we are displacing, not replacing. The focus here, at this point, is to highlight the keto items in your meals.

Think of it this way. You're in a big space, it's dark, and then there's a spotlight. There are several food items in the middle of the space. Instead of shining the spotlight on all the food items, shine it only on the keto items.

Now, this means that you're not cutting out all the other foods on your meal plan. You're just emphasizing, as far as your attention and your taste buds go, the keto-friendly items.

This is how you prepare yourself for the scale-down process. Otherwise, it's easy to just hit a plateau. Seriously.

I've seen this happen. Of the people who transitioned from the standard American diet to a keto diet, many keep hitting this wall. They can't let go of the other foods because they focus on all the items on their meal plans.

You must start looking forward to the keto items. You must start celebrating their taste profiles. Get yourself excited about these foods more than the diet.

This is a key change in your mindset because a lot of people who are pumped up about the keto diet are pumped up about the weight loss.

Let's be completely honest here. They couldn't really care less about the taste. A lot actually have misgivings, but they are excited about finally getting rid of that nasty spare tire they've been lugging around in their midsection since what seems like forever.

Believe me, I understand where these individuals are coming from. But until and unless you get excited about the food itself, instead of the diet or what you could get from the diet, you're going to have a tough time.

There, I said it.

Sure, you may lose quite a bit of weight. It may seem, at least from the outside, that you're doing well. But eventually, something will get knocked loose. It's only a matter of time until you go back to your old eating patterns because you focus on all the items in your meal plan.

Unfortunately, not all of them are keto-friendly. This is why it's really important to get used to eating keto foods and highlight them or focus on them more when you eat.

When you're looking forward to your next meal, get excited about the keto food items. Do this for several days, if not weeks, and then you will be ready for the scale-down process.

Start to Scale Down Your Carb Intake Dramatically

Please understand that our goal here is to trigger ketosis by using this diet. This involves a transition phase. But eventually, you must be fully ketogenic.

In other words, at a certain point in time, you must flip over to using fat as your main energy source instead of sugar. This is the point where things get real with the keto diet.

All the previous chapters that I've walked you through prepare you for this point in time. This can only happen when you start to scale down your carb intake dramatically.

How come? As I have mentioned in a previous chapter, if insulin is in the picture, you're not burning fat for fuel. Seriously. It really is that simple.

If you eat more than 12 to 25 carb grams every single day, your body will be producing insulin and you're mostly burning sugar throughout the day for energy.

At this point in time, you're going to have to scale down your carb intake dramatically so you can get below the 12 to 25-gram maximum daily carb intake threshold.

Thankfully, there are two wonder foods that you can rely on to get you there.

Your Keto Wonder Food #1: Eggs

I don't know about you, but I've always had a softness for eggs. They're compact, they're pretty straightforward, they're definitely easy to prepare, and they are loaded with nutrition.

Eggs are packed with all sorts of vitamins and nutrients, and they really don't pack much calories on a gram per gram basis.

Did you know that Weight Watchers no longer give points for eggs? If you don't know the Weight Watcher system, when you eat certain food items, you are given points. And you can only eat so much food until you hit a certain point threshold.

If you go over that maximum point threshold, you're going to gain weight. If you eat below it, you lose weight.

For the longest time, Weight Watchers was giving eggs points. Well, they've wiped those points out. Now, you can basically eat quite a bit of eggs.

This is in keeping with recent research that shows that eggs are not bad for you. For the longest time, eggs were demonized in the United States and elsewhere as these cholesterol bombs.

Well, it turns out, after decades of research, that it's sugar that is making us sick and fat. Not eggs. And definitely not dietary fat. Interesting how things change, right?

This is why it's a good idea to load up on eggs. Maybe you like them boiled, maybe you like them sunny side up, it doesn't matter. Load up on eggs. This is a great keto food.

One to two eggs should be fine. They fill you up and they make you feel fuller for a longer period of time.

Your Keto Wonder Food #2: Avocado

As I've mentioned earlier, avocado is not exactly a "default taste" for most people. It's not like you wake up one day and you just say, "I can't wait to enjoy a plain avocado." That rarely happens.

Either you eat avocado in the form of ice cream, or you turn it into guacamole. But as a fruit by itself, added into a salad of greens, that takes some doing. It definitely takes some getting used to. My wife and I actually enjoy it as an ingredient to our salads.

But if you really want to take your keto diet to the next level and scale down your carb intake dramatically, load up on avocado. It's loaded in fat, but it also has dietary fiber and is loaded with vitamins. It's really good for you.

And it is actually easy to get used to because it's very versatile. You can mix it with all sorts of greens. You can mix it with egg. It's good stuff. One of the latest ways to enjoy it is to make a paste out of it and spread it on toast; you may have heard of avocado toast? That's it!

Your Keto Wonder Food #3: Cauliflower

I include cauliflower here knowing full well that it does have carbohydrates. This is why it's a good idea to use moderate amounts of cauliflower. Maybe you can prepare it once every other day, or a little more frequently.

I include cauliflower here because a lot of us veterans of the standard American diet are used to eating a significant amount of carbohydrates every day. In my case, I used to eat a lot of rice.

Cauliflower saved my life as far as my keto diet goes. Why? Instead of loading up on brown rice, red rice, or plain steamed white rice, I make cauliflower "rice." You just grind it up and then you fry it.

You can turn it into "fried rice" or you can serve it plain fried or sautéed. It has roughly the same consistency as rice, but it's loaded with protein instead of carbs.

Of course, you should only eat a moderate amount of protein daily. You can't go overboard with protein because, as I have mentioned earlier in this book, your liver actually turns protein into sugar. This is called glucogenesis.

You don't want this to happen because you want to minimize the amount of sugar, regardless of its source, in your system for ketosis to work its wonders.

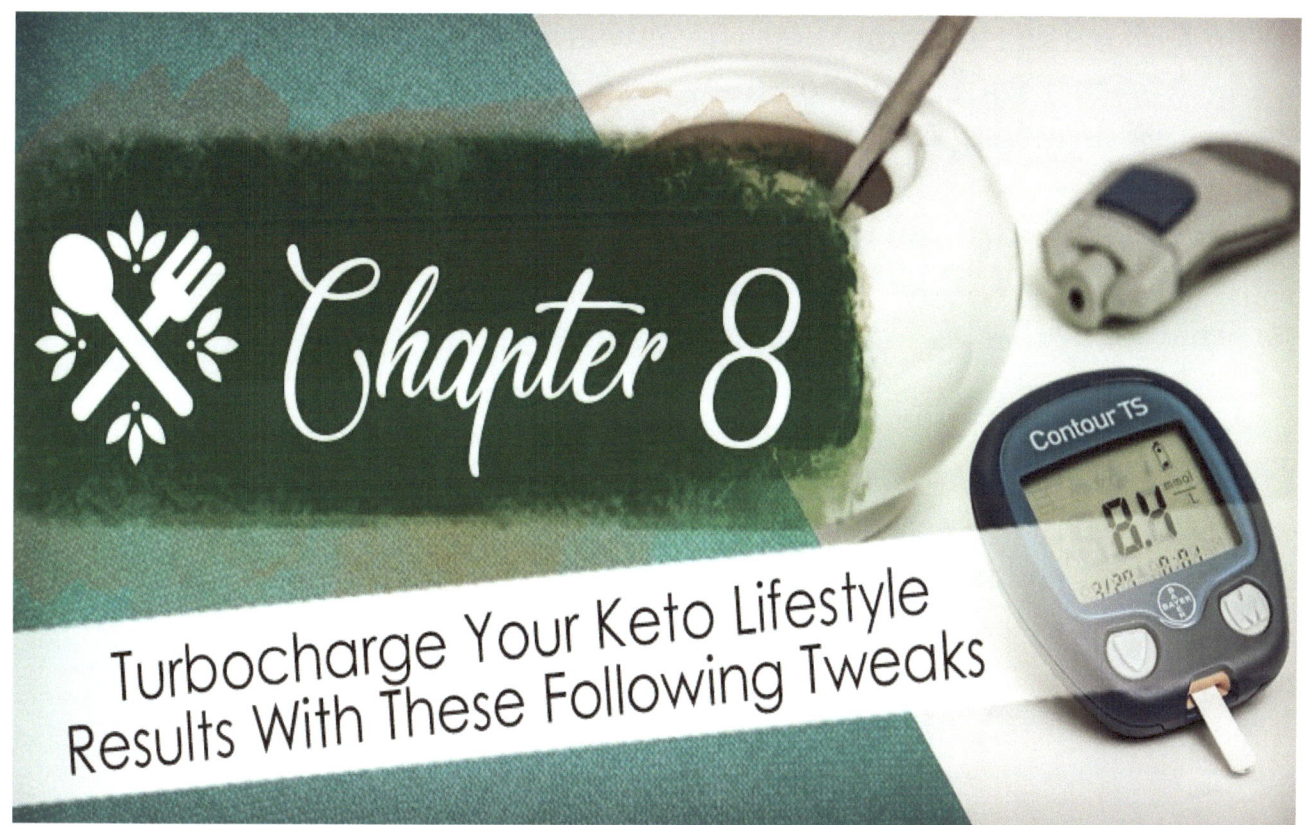

Chapter 8 – Turbocharge Your Keto Lifestyle Result With These Following Tweaks

I'm not going to lie to you, switching to a new diet can be very challenging. It definitely will take quite a bit of effort. It definitely requires a lot of focus and willpower – that is the part where having the right mindset comes in.

And if you want to stick to a diet and keep the pounds off indefinitely, you're going to have to focus on consistency; this is your diet for the rest of your life.

Thankfully, there are certain tweaks that would enable you to convert your keto diet into a keto lifestyle. This really is the secret to any kind of weight loss program.

If you look at diet just as a means for you to lose a few pounds here and there, then chances are, you're going to regain those pounds. It's only a matter of time.

If you look back at all of the diets you have tried in the past, this was probably your experience with them too – they were never meant to be a lifestyle ... only for a short-term loss.

On the other hand, if you look at your weight loss system as a gateway or a transition point to a different lifestyle, then the weight is probably going to stay off. That's how it works.

Keep the following tweaks in mind. I don't expect you to master all of these the first time you try them. Usually, it takes a while to get used to them, but eventually, they will become second nature to you as long as you give them enough focus and importance.

Eat Only When You're Hungry

I can't even begin to tell you how many people eat out of obligation, boredom or when under emotional or physical stress. I know that sounds crazy. It definitely sounds ridiculous, but it's true.

I know it because it happened to me. This was my standard practice. I would look at my watch or my mobile phone and notice that it's a certain time. That's when I know it's time to eat.

So, regardless of whether I'm hungry, or regardless of how busy I am, I just sit down and enjoy my meal. That's a serious problem.

Because if you're not hungry, you don't have to take in those calories. You can just lose yourself in your work or you can just focus on what you're doing regardless of the time.

It doesn't matter what your schedule is, if you're not hungry, you don't have to eat.

This is a hard habit to break. A lot of this has to do with our upbringing. Our parents, bless them, would sit us down at certain fixed times.

In my household, we were expected to eat from 6 to 7:30 a.m., and then from 11 to 12:30 p.m. Our final meal together would be from 6 to 8:00 p.m., depending on people's schedules. But those are the time ranges.

When you've been doing that for many years, it's hard to break free. It's hard to try something new. It's as if your body clock has essentially evolved around those schedules.

But there's really no rule written on granite stone that dictates that you should eat out of obligation because of time.

If you want to convert your keto diet into a lifestyle that you can stick to for life, eat only when you're hungry. This is the most empowering thing you can do.

You're eating to live. You're not living to eat. I know that sounds like a cliché (and it is), but it's also true.

You're not eating out of obligation. You're not eating out of custom or tradition. You're not eating because "that's just what I do."

No. You're eating because you want to. And you should only want to eat because you're feeling hungry.

Drink First When You Get Hunger Pangs

It's very easy to just go to a drive-thru or to the nearest restaurant or even a corner grocery store and buy some ready-made meal when you feel hunger pangs. After all, you are hungry. You're doing something to take care of the hunger as soon as possible.

I get that. That's what most people do.

The problem is, the hunger that you're feeling may not linger for long. Those hunger pangs may be temporary. If fact, you may just be thirsty.

41

The signs are similar to hunger pangs.

This is why I suggest that you drink first when you get hunger pangs. You'd be surprised as to how quickly your hunger dissipates.

The secret here is to drink first. Now, don't go crazy. There's no need to go overboard. You don't have to whip out a liter of water or a gallon jug and start pounding away.

No. Just a small cup would do. See if it does the trick. And then have another glass.

Another trick that I use is to first drink warm water. If you can get it, drink a little bit of hot water. You'd be surprised as to how much of your hunger pangs is actually just your body looking to rehydrate itself.

Stick to this plan: drink first when you get hunger pangs, drink warm water first, then drink more cold water. If that doesn't do the trick, then decide to eat.

Eat Slowly

Once you have decided to eat, don't rush through the process. I know, this is easier said than done.

If you're like most Americans, you feel that you really don't have much time. In fact, if you're like most people, you'd think that time is a luxury. Believe me, I understand where you're coming from and I totally get you.

But here's the thing. If you just blow through your meal, your mind is not going to register satiety fully. It will still be partly hungry.

So, what do you think happens next? That's right. You eat even more calories until you're finally sated. Usually, in that context, your body only feels full when your stomach has expanded enough.

As you can well imagine, this is not a recipe for weight loss. You end up eating too much. This is why it's a good idea to eat slowly.

You're eating your keto meals. That's awesome. But eat slowly.

This means that you get to enjoy your food more. It also gives your brain time to synchronize and line up with your body.

Because when you eat, you're actually releasing chemical compounds through your body. It's sending all sorts of signals. There's this interplay between your brain and the rest of your body, particularly your digestive tract.

If you rush through your meals, this delicate balance of signals cascading into each other and reacting to each other doesn't play out fully. So, you end up overloading your system with calories.

Eat slowly. There's no rush. Enjoy each mouthful. Celebrate your food.

Again, eat to live. Don't live to eat.

Look at Each of Your Meals as Some Sort of Event

When you have chosen to eat slowly, your mind has opened itself to the possibility of looking at food as some sort of celebration. It is not just empty generic fuel that you just load up on so you can do more important things throughout the day.

Unfortunately, this is how most people view food.

Food is an end in and of itself. It is something to be celebrated. It is part of what makes life special. You need to slow down and eat more deliberately for you to really savor your food.

Once you've started to do that, then eventually, you will be able to look at your meals as some sort of event. It's something to look forward to.

It's kind of like your feast for the day.

Eat More Mindfully

Not only should you eat slowly, but you should also be as conscious of the eating process as possible.

Savor each mouthful. Be aware of the flavors going through your mouth. Understand yourself more fully by experiencing your food preferences in a more direct way.

Different people have different tastes. Different people have different preferences. When you eat more mindfully, the meals say something about you.

They say something about your preference. They say something about the textures that you like. They are part of an event. You're connected to the whole eating process.

When you eat, choose to eat. In other words, focus your attention on what you're doing.

It is no surprise that a lot of people who are multitasking while they're eating tend to eat too much. They also tend to eat more frequently.

How come? They're not there. Their attention is somewhere else.

Maybe it's in the email that they're monitoring or maybe it's in the social media updates that are obsessed about, or maybe it's work. Maybe they're talking to other people. Whatever the case may be, they are not letting the eating process unwind itself.

You have to understand that, just like sleep, eating is a big part of you. All people must eat. It doesn't matter what corner of the globe you come from, it doesn't matter what your specific background is, you must eat if you are a member of the human species.

It really is a tragedy that you go through your meals like it's an afterthought. You have to pack as much meaning into it like you would with sleep.

One third of your life is spent sleeping. Well, a significant portion is also spent eating. Wouldn't it be great if you're more aware and appreciative of that percentage of your precious time you spend eating?

The good news is that this will pay off handsomely when it comes to weight loss. You'll be able to keep the weight off because you don't have to eat as much. And also, when you're eating keto foods, you enjoy them better and they make you feel fuller for a longer period of time.

Chapter 9 - Take Things to the Next Level With These Modifications

Prior to this point, all the tips, tricks and tweaks that I've shared with you can help you maximize the effects of ketosis. They will help you flip the script from using blood sugar as your main energy source to burning fat.

You probably have already lost quite a number of pounds prior to this point. So far, so good. But if you are serious about taking things to the next level, focus on the following modifications.

Please understand that these modifications are not easy. It's a good idea to master all the previous chapters first.

Lock them down. Know them backwards and forwards. Incorporate them into your lifestyle. Get used to them.

Once things have gotten "easy" and you've totally gotten used to the previous modifications, now is the time to level up.

Start to Regularize Your Mealtimes

You need to start giving yourself certain rules regarding your meals. If you notice that there is a certain pattern for your hunger cycles, get them down in writing. Try to regularize them.

The key here is to strike a deal with yourself. If you don't eat within these fixed regular times where you're normally hungry, you resolve not to eat at all until the next period.

This is a big break for a lot of people. But once you get over this hump, the fat, seriously, just melts off. It's unbelievable because you reduce your calorie intake quite a bit.

And the best part is that once you get used to this, you don't even miss those calories. This is because you have resolved to know your hunger patterns and internal body clock schedule intimately.

This takes quite a bit of self-awareness. This definitely takes quite a bit of time and effort. It's not like you know these already.

Because a lot of people with shifting schedules are very distracted. It turns out that their bodies actually have fairly fixed hunger cycles, but they wouldn't know it because they are focused on their other schedules.

They're focused on their work schedule. They're focused on going to and from their home. But once you zero in on your hunger cycles and you regularize these in terms of your mealtimes, you make quite a bit of progress.

Because eventually, you would be able to skip meals if you're not feeling hungry within a specific period of time. And then you would be able to wait until you're hungry again for the next period.

Also, your mind gets used to it and you are able to stick to your meal times.

Eliminate or Greatly Reduce Snacking

Prior to this point, you can still snack. But eventually, once you've regularized your mealtimes and your hunger cycles become more controlled and fixed, you can start eliminating snacking.

Now, please understand that this is not going to happen overnight.

You've probably been snacking all your life. Welcome to the club. That's how most people are. That's perfectly okay.

But once you have a good hold or control over your hunger schedule, you can make amazing progress in greatly reducing or flat out eliminating snacking.

I know it seems like a pipe dream right now. It seems almost impossible. But you'd be surprised as to what you're capable of if you put your mind to it.

Start with a gradual reduction. It doesn't have to be big. You don't have to be a hero. You're not looking for some sort of great leap ahead. You just want to make a little change.

You'd be surprised as to how quickly you can do this because you've taken the right initial steps, which is to regularize your mealtimes.

Eventually Scale Down to Two Meals a Day

I have to admit, if I were to tell this to you upfront, it will probably set you back. You probably would be thinking, "No, this guy is crazy. This is not going to happen. I eat regularly, I eat three square meals a day, with a few snacks in between."

Believe me, I understand where you're coming from because that was my mindset.

But once I was able to regularize my mealtimes and I was able to practice everything else in this book prior to this point, this was the eventual conclusion. Seriously. This is where you're headed.

Because if you did everything that I've told you correctly, this is where you will be. You will be able to scale down to one or two meals a day.

Obviously, you're going to scale down to two. Then once that gets easy and predictable, scale down to one.

Now, why is this a big deal? Even if you load up on food on that one meal a day, you still cut out a tremendous number of calories from your diet.

If you also adopt some sort of modest exercise program, this can go a long way in burning the fat off.

By modest exercise, I'm not talking about you running a marathon. There's no need to do that. You don't have to become some sort of triathlete or fancy yourself as some sort of ironman or ironwoman. No need to be a hero, once again.

You can just walk around the block or you can bike around. It doesn't matter. Any kind of moderate exercise is enough to tip the scales, especially when you've reduced everything down to one to two meals a day.

Scale Down to One Meal a Day

In this section, I want to make it clear that this is not you going down to one meal every once in a while. This is not you going down to one meal a day, three times a week. Instead, this is you scaling down to one meal a day as an iron rule.

Now, this might seem a bit hard. And it is for a lot of people. But if you followed all the steps above, it's easier to get to this point than you care to imagine.

You've laid the groundwork, so making the transition is not really as abrupt and as hard as you think. What's important here is that when you decide to eat only once a day, it must be a commitment.

The deal is this: you choose to eat only within a certain time window. This is called intermittent fasting paired with a keto diet.

When you make this deal with yourself, this means that if you go past the window, you're going to skip the meal. You wait until the next day.

That may seem harsh, but when I started this, I was shocked at how easy it was because I would go by a whole day forgetting that I actually did not eat anything for the whole day. That's how natural it felt once you reach that point.

That's the secret to intermittent fasting. It's a commitment to eat within a certain time frame.

You need to be on the same page with your primary care physician. Any advice here that I give you must be run through and approved by your doctor.

If you engage in any kind of fasting, make sure you talk with your doctor first. Still, when you adopt intermittent fasting, it really turbocharges your weight loss and it exaggerates the weight loss effects of the keto diet.

If You Can, Adopt a Day to Day Fasting Technique

This is really taking things to the next level. With a day to day fasting technique, you're basically eating within a certain time window one day, and then completely avoiding any food the next day, and then going back to eating.

Now, a lot of people never reach this point. This is purely optional. But if you want to really level things up, this is definitely a good candidate.

Some people even take things to a whole other level. They would go two days fasting, and then three days eating, and then back to two days fasting.

That may be too extreme, but it's definitely an option you should explore once you're able to pull off all the other steps described above.

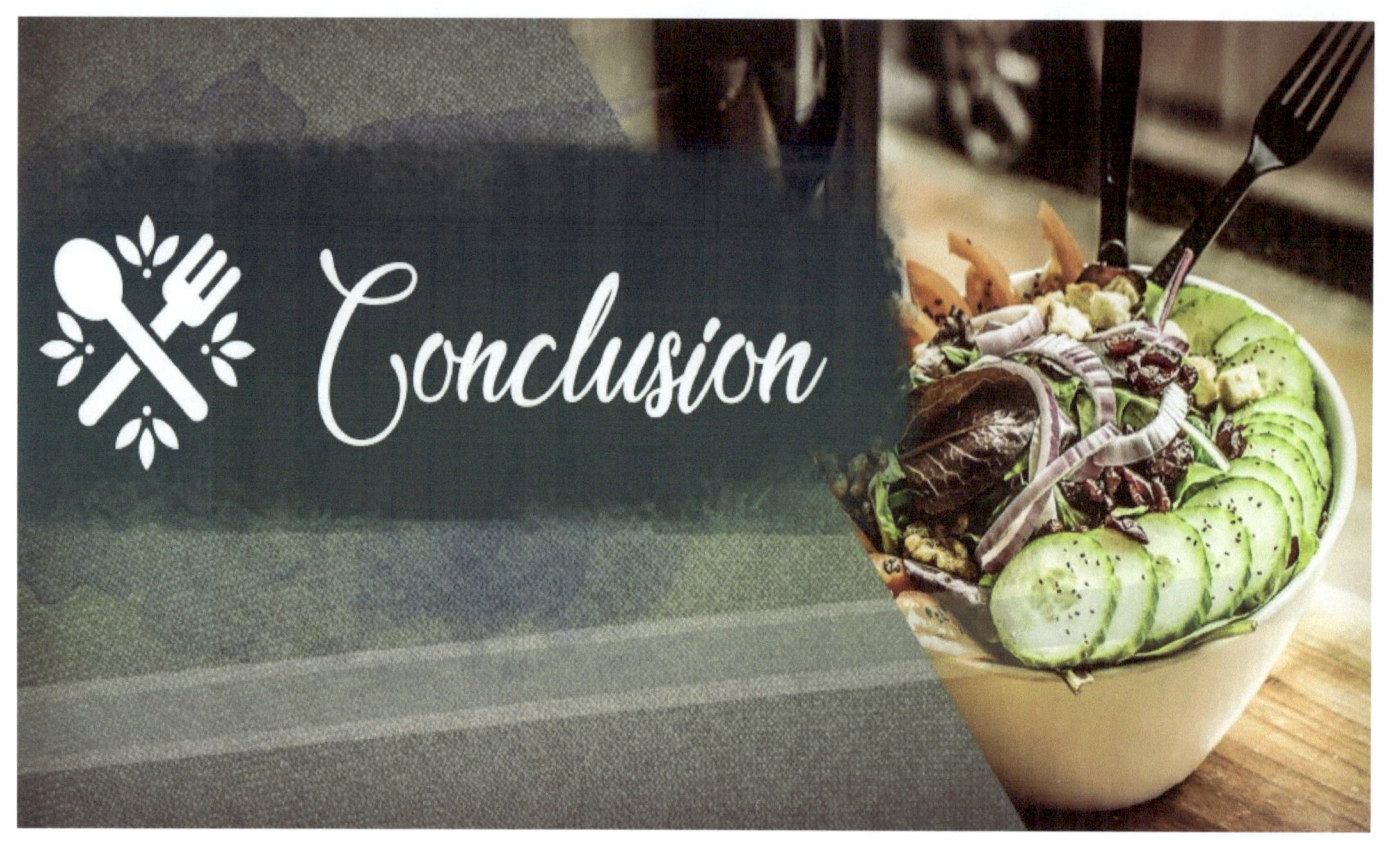

Conclusion

The keto diet is achievable. How do I know? Well, I've done it. And before I started, other people have done it before me. Currently at the time of this writing, it is one of the hottest diets among celebrities and athletes alike. It is the diet used by LeBron James, Koby Bryant, Tim McGraw, Halle Berry and Gwyneth Paltrow, Mick Jagger, Drew Carey ... just to name a few. Just search the Internet and you will find all kinds of famous people that have had and are currently having success with this diet. If it works for them and their busy life, it will work for you. After all, what do you have to lose?

I want you to wrap your mind around that. This is not something impossible. This is not something outlandish or out of this world. You can eat fatty foods that you've enjoyed for a long time and not feel guilty about it.

Instead of worrying about your waistline, fat can actually be the secret ingredient that would help you melt those pounds away. I know, it is counter-intuitive to everything you have done in the past. But has the past worked for you?

Most likely not or you wouldn't be here now!

I don't care how long you've been carrying that nasty looking spare tire around your midsection. With the right focus, mindset, implementation and attention to detail, the keto diet will make that fat go away ... for good!

The good news is, if other people can do it, you can do it too. But here's the key: don't look at it as yet another diet.

If you've gone from diet to diet with very little permanent change, you'll be in for a surprise. If you look at the keto diet as an invitation to changing your overall lifestyle to one that is healthy, then you are less likely to go back to your old eating habits.

If you need help keeping on this Keto diet, may I suggest my 21-Day Bulletproof Keto Diet Workbook. You can purchase it at:
https://www.amazon.com/dp/1070519529.

Why 21 days? That is usually how long it takes to engrain a new eating plan into a habit. Once it is a habit, it is easier to stick to it, but some people need a resource they can use that will help them get to the habit point. This workbook does just that.

I wish you nothing but the greatest success.

The Keto Diet Cheat Sheet

Your Goal: Burn More Fat Passively by eating fat. How? Use fat as your body's fuel instead of sugar!

The objective? Achieving ketosis = Burning fat instead of sugar

Step 1: Resolve to change your lifestyle instead of yet going on another diet:

- Think long term
- Believe that the keto lifestyle works
- Believe that you can do it
- If other people can do it, you can do it too

Step 2: Displace, not replace"

- Add keto items to your diet
- Gradually get away from your old eating habits and focus more on ketogenic meals

Step 3: Make the following meal plan choices:

- Focus on fatty food that fits your taste
- Shoot to feel fuller for a longer period of time after eating
- Eventually cut out all soda
- Eventually cut out all grain-based snacks
- Slowly cut out milk-based snacks

Step 4: Wind down carbs:

- By this point, you have gotten used to eating keto foods
- Start to scale down your carb intake dramatically
- Eat more eggs
- Eat more avocados

Step 5: Step up keto weight loss with the following new habits:

- Eat only when you're hungry
- Drink first when you get hunger pangs
- Eat slowly
- Look at each of your meals as some sort of event
- Eat more mindfully

Step 6: Finetune your keto diet:

- Start to regularize your meal times
- Eliminate or greatly reduce snacking
- Eventually scale down to one or two meals a day
- Scale down to one meal a day: intermittent fasting
- If you can, adopt a day-to-day fasting technique

The Bulletproof Keto Diet Resources

Resource #1

Daily Nutrient Inventory:

- To the best of your ability, record all the food you ate today
- Break them down into the following categories
  - Fat (must be 85% of your total calories)
  - Carbohydrates (limit: 10 to 20 grams)
  - Protein (no more than 10 to 12% of your total calories)

Goal: Maximize your fat intake and sustain it.

Resource #2

Meal Type Time Tracker:

- Note (https://www.amazon.com/gp/product/1541392868) down the nutrient type of your meal (mostly fat, mostly protein, mostly carbs)
- Note down the time of your meal

Goal: Space out the times so you feel fuller for a longer period of time – this also decreases your total calorie intake.

Resource #3

Brainstorm the different ways you can prepare eggs:

- Eat eggs every day
- Prepare eggs in a different way

Goal: Eat more eggs without getting bored.

Resource #4

List potential Keto "Accountability Buddies":

- Write down all the people you know who are doing keto
- Talk to them about being accountability buddies
- Share with them resources 1 to 3 above
- Keep tabs on each other

Goal: Encourage each other to stay on track with the keto diet.

Resource #5

Routine Tracking:

- Write down your most consistent daily routine
- Which parts of your routine can you change so you stay keto?

Goal: Keep mixing things up until you get the right combination that works for you.

If you would like to learn even more about the keto diet, here is another resource to consider: https://www.amazon.com/gp/product/B07NQ2Z67X

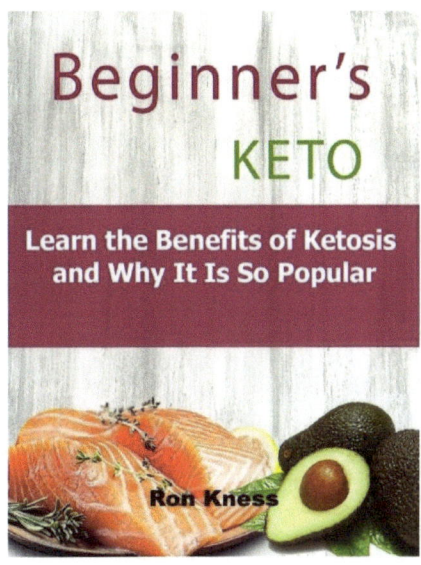

About the Author

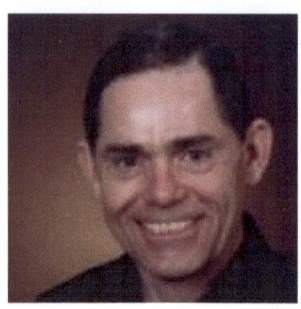

I have published numerous books both digital and printed on Amazon for Kindle and other publishing platforms including Draft2Digital and Lulu.

While most of my books are on health and fitness in general, as I age my topics of interest are geared toward aging baby boomers and the older generation and some of their unique health issues, such as weight gain.

Besides my own writing, I also ghostwrite ebooks, POD books, reports, articles, blogs and do Kindle conversions for clients on a variety of topics.

Today my wife and I are retired from our careers and live in San Tan Valley, AZ. I now write as a retirement business where you'll find me happily sitting in my office typing away on my laptop as I work on my next book or ghostwriting project . . . that is if we are not traveling on a cruise ship - our new-found mode of travel.